Customer Service Training
for
Healthcare Professionals

Improve your customer service practices

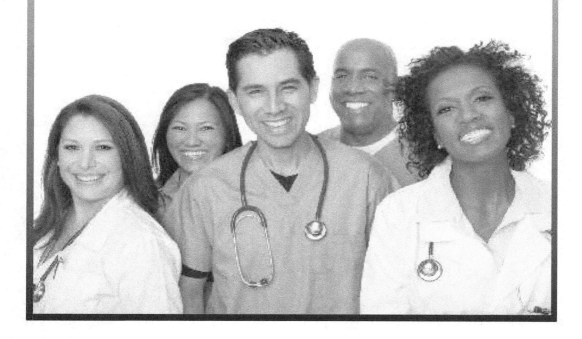

Customer Service for Healthcare Professionals

Customer Service Training for Healthcare Professionals

Request for information should be addressed to the author or publisher

Insight Consulting International Group
Dr. Reba Haley
P.O Box 648
Valrico, Florida 33595

Reba Haley – Customer Service for Healthcare Professionals

Library of Congress cataloging in publication Library of Congress cataloging in publication data Haley, Reba Library of Congress

Customer Service Training for Healthcare Professionals

Insight Consulting International Group, Inc.
Website: icigroupintl.org
Email: icigintl@gmail.com

ISBN 9-780964659445

Customer Service for Healthcare Professionals

Customer Service for Healthcare Professionals

TABLE OF CONTENTS

Customer Service for Healthcare Professionals

Introduction

Customer Service Training for Healthcare Professionals is written in English and Spanish for students and interns that are entering the healthcare workforce and employees that work with patients in long-term care facilities, hospitals, or clinics. According to the Department of Labor," employment of healthcare occupations is projected to grow 18% from 2018 to 2026 much faster than the average for all occupations, adding about 2.4 million new jobs." Also, the Bureau of Labor and Statistics reports that healthcare is the largest employer in the United States.

Customer Service Training for Healthcare Professionals provides students and interns and employees with customer services principles and communication strategies to improve patient treatment outcomes and patient relations. In healthcare, patient care is the most critical factor yet regularly healthcare professionals overlook customer service. In today's healthcare industry employers are looking for people with excellent customer service. Healthcare is a business and employers want people to provide the best care to their patients. Often time's healthcare professionals overlook patients as customers; however, patients differ from other customers, in that they don't want to be ill or, a customer. The physician's office or hospital experience can be scary and confusing for patients. The book helps you learn how to provide excellent customer service, demonstrate professional workplace

Customer Service for Healthcare Professionals

behaviors, achieve patient satisfaction, display empathy, and provide quality patient care. *Customer Service Training for Healthcare Professionals* will help you improve your listening and communication skills. Active listening and proper documentation can help you prevent medical errors and improve patient care. In today's, healthcare industry superior customer service is critical in retaining patients and attracting new ones. A study suggested that the longer patients wait to be seen by a healthcare professional, the more the patient satisfaction rate drops. In healthcare, you will encounter various types of customer behaviors, complaints, and problems. Understanding personality types and actions can help you work with people from diverse cultures and ethnicities without offending patients. You will become aware of your cultural heritage, attitude, and belief and prejudices and learn to value and respect differences. Increased knowledge and awareness of culturally different patients/customers can build culturally competent healthcare professionals.

Customer Service Training for Healthcare Professionals is uniquely designed for healthcare professionals to develop essential skills to improve customer service and create positive patient experiences. The goals are to improve customer service, increase patient satisfaction, enhance internal and external communication skills, and create positive, memorable experiences for patients and families.

Best Wishes

Reba

Customer Service for Healthcare Professionals

Chapter 1

Customer Service in Healthcare

Customer Service training in healthcare is an investment and organizations, schools and healthcare professionals can benefit from workplace training tools. In-service training or professional training in customer service allows employees and students to improve their human interaction skills. Training will enable people who work with the public to conduct a self-assessment and identify areas that need improvement. Professional training allows participants to recognize their prejudices and biases. Often training is necessary to change behaviors of prejudices, biases, stereotyping attitudes and prejudgments.

Healthcare professionals should focus on providing superior customer service and patient care. From the moment the patient enters the healthcare facility they make a judgment about the facility and you. Greeting customers are essential in building a good impression. Body language and tone of voice creates a customer's first impression. Excellent customer service starts by first getting to know the patient and showing that he /she are essential.

Scheduling appointments properly and avoiding long wait lines can improve customer satisfaction. Providing excellent quality customer service is crucial in healthcare. Greeting customers and meeting their needs and concerns create a strong first impression. Providing excellent customer service, listening and communicating appropriate can make patients/customers advocates. Effective communication such as; telephone, face to face interactions, emailing and faxing are essential customer service skills in healthcare. The lack of communication can cause misunderstandings and medical errors.

The Joint Commission accredits and certifies more than 20,500 health care organizations and programs in the United States. Joint Commission accreditation and certification is recognized nationwide as a symbol of quality that reflects an organization's commitment to meeting certain performance standards. According to the Joint Commission, if medical errors appeared on the National Center for Health Statistic's list of the top 10 causes of death in the United States, they would rank number 5—ahead of accidents, diabetes, and Alzheimer's disease, as well as AIDS, breast cancer, and gunshot wounds. Even more disturbing, communication failures are the leading root cause of the sentinel events reported from 1995 to 2004. The Joint Commission 2015 report, wrong-patient errors occurred in virtually all stages of diagnosis and treatment.

More specifically, the Joint Commission cites communication failures as the leading root cause for medication errors, delays in treatment, and wrong-site surgeries, as well as the second most frequently cited root cause for operative and postoperative events and fatal falls. In 2015 the Joint Commission goal was to improve the accuracy of patient identification. (www.jointcommission.org)

One of the most critical concerns in healthcare is patient identification, and healthcare facilities have implemented a patient identification system to avoid medical errors.

How to Avoid Medical Errors

1. Don't Rush- Take Your Time
2. Develop a matching patient system
3. Identity patients by name and match to wristbands
4. Develop an alphabetic or chronological medical records filing system
5. Ask patients their name and date of birth and match the patient to the chart and room number
6. When transferring patients, verify the patient's name, room number and wristband.

According to the Joint Commission accurately identifying patients and careful planning before medical treatment can provide safer care for patients and significantly decrease medical errors. Verifying the patient's name accurately and effective communication can prevent medical errors. The Joint Commission recommended the use of two identifiers such as; name and date of birth to verify a patient's identity upon admission or transfer to another hospital or other healthcare settings, and before the administration of care. They also recommended if the patient is in the hospital that the patient's room number be used to identify the patient.

Healthcare professionals work with people from diverse cultures and ethnicities and working with people from different backgrounds can make healthcare workers more sensitive. The lack of cultural awareness can affect treatment outcomes and patient care. Competent healthcare workers identify their prejudices and biases and acknowledge cultural differences. Healthcare is a business, and effective communication is essential when working with internal and external consumer/customers. Effective communication is central to breaking down barriers, eliminating fears and improving interactions with patients. Communicating can help you get to know your patient, prevent injuries, build trust, and improve patient and provider relationship.

The goals of healthcare professionals are to provide quality patient care, create positive patient experiences, and ensure customer satisfaction. One of the most effective ways to greet a customer is by addressing them by Mr, Miss or Mrs (name). Greeting customers with a smile and greeting them by name displays friendliness and approachability. Welcoming patients/customers can have a positive impact on healthcare and make patients/customers feel valued.

Greeting customers are the first impression of your service quality and can make patients feel welcomed. Demonstrating professional workplace behaviors and communicating appropriate are essential in building good working relationships with patients.

Exceptional Customer Service

Identifying and determining a patient/customer need helps a healthcare professional provide proper medical care. In healthcare providers will come in contact with demanding patients/customers. However, it is essential to provide good customer service and patient care to everyone. Excellent customer service can create patient satisfaction and attract new patients. Customer service surveys and discharge surveys help office managers and medical administrators determine what changes are needed to improve patient care. Customer service satisfaction surveys are useful in collecting and critical to monitoring patient's quality of care.

Core Customer Service Beliefs

The ten customer service core beliefs are the foundation for building exceptional customer service in the healthcare industry. These are the foundations that you can continually do and build on.

1. Customers are valued and vital people, whether they are in person, on the phone or by mail.

2. Customers deserve outstanding service. It is our responsibilities to provide care in a manner that is mutually beneficial and with satisfactory results.

3. Customers are not an interruption to your job. They are the reason that you have a job.

4. Customers must not feel dependent on us, but on the contrary, we are dependent on them.

5. Customers are people like us, not numbers, or statistics.

6. Customers are not people to argue, challenge, humiliated or embarrassed. Customers are to be treated with dignity and respect.

7. Customers have a right to receive prompt and courteous service, regardless of their culture or behavior.

8. Customers are part of what we do, not people on the outside.

9. Customers provide us with opportunities to serve them. When patients are engaged in their healthcare, it can lead to a working partnership.

10. Customers have the same expectations as we do when we are in the role of a customer.

Enhanced customer service standards can improve employee performance and customer satisfaction. Customers expect employees who work with patients to be professional and caring. A patient wants to know what you can do and will do for them to make them feel better.

Customer Service for Healthcare Professionals

A healthcare professional should speak to a customer in a tone and manner that is positive and helpful. The words you choose and your tone of voice tells a customer if you want to help them or not.

Showing kindness is the first step you show customers that they are valued, and you want to help them. Research suggests that compassion can lead to faster healing and positive treatment outcomes. Healthcare professionals should demonstrate messages of respect on the telephone and face-to-face.

Here are some words and phrases that can help you create a positive impression and show customers/ patients that you care.

_____

_____

_____

_____

_____

Customer Service for Healthcare Professionals

Command Words to Avoid	Desire Words to Say
<ul><li>You have to</li><li>You can't</li><li>We can't</li><li>I don't know</li><li>Have to,</li><li>Go to</li><li>Expect to</li><li>Need to</li><li>Suppose to</li><li>Blame You</li><li>Obligate you</li><li>Deserve to</li></ul>	<ul><li>I would like to</li><li>Here are some suggestions</li><li>I am unable to but, I will find out</li><li>I would like</li><li>It would be best</li><li>I suggest</li><li>I would be nice</li><li>I would rather.</li></ul>

According to the Webster dictionary, the health professional is "an individual who provides preventive, curative, promotional, or rehabilitative health care services in a systematic way to people, families, or communities." A person seeking medical attention could be a patient, coworker, and superior. Most people see health professional as experts. Treating patients with respect and dignity will improve the patient and healthcare relationship. Again noted, research suggests patients that feel respected can have favorable treatment. A patient's that feels you care about them will open up and talk about his or her medical concerns. Greeting customers in a friendly and helpful manner create trust.

Customer Service Skills

Greet customers with a smile	Convey a willingness to help
Hear and remember the significant customer concerns	Anticipate the needs and have an answer prepared
Express appreciation from external, internal customers	Make customers feel important
Follow up with the customer	Do your best to handle and manage problems and concerns quickly
Show dignity and respect	Give customer useful information
Communicate clear and concise	Be friendly and kind
Use positive words	Summarize customers' needs and interests

Pair up with someone else and role-play and give an example of a positive and negative customer healthcare scenario. Include diverse cultures to promote cultural sensitivity service scenario.

Cultural Diversity in Healthcare

Cultural Competence is the ability to respond effectively and appropriately to different cultural/generational contexts in the workplace.

- Acknowledge and accept differences
- Seek to understand; ask for clarification or reasons for the behavior
- Respect others' opinions.
- Be open to learning about other cultures and ideas.
- Give others the benefit of the doubt in a dispute.

With the increase in diverse groups and differences in culture and religious beliefs in America, healthcare professionals should be culturally competent and aware of cultural differences. Cultural incompetence can lead to inappropriate treatment and poor treatment outcomes.

1. We are diverse in many ways, including race, gender, age, education, cultural background, and physical abilities. True or False

2. Diversity is a way to encourage new ideas and perspectives. True or False

3. We are diverse in many ways, including race, gender, age, education,   cultural background, and physical abilities. True or False

Chapter 2

Caring for Your Customer

Patients don't want to feel that they are just a name but that they are unique and valued customers. Everyone wants to feel valued and showing customers that you care will go a long way. The way you treat patients shows professionalism. A demonstration of interest and concern are indicators that you care for your patient/customer. Researchers suggest that one satisfied customer will share their experience with twenty people. If customers feel that you care about them, they will refer other people to your healthcare facility. The acronym CARE is the characteristics and qualities of healthcare professionals.

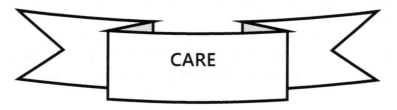

Credibility - your credibility is critical in the healthcare industry. When you show the patient that you can, it reinforces that they are valued.

Active voice- communicating in a pleasant tone and attentive listening shows the customers that you care.

Customer Service for Healthcare Professionals

Retention- being reliable in meeting the patients/customers' needs and addressing their concern creates loyal customers.

Empathy- see every patient/customer as unique and go out of your way to solve their problems, it will create a customer for life.

Caring for the customer means that you communicate and show interest in their wellness and that you care about them on a personal level.

Caring for the customer means that you provide personalized service to create a positive customer experience. Take your customer service skills to the next level and improve your communication and personalization skills.

Strengthening your communication skills and improving your personalization skills are essential aspects of providing quality healthcare and superior customer service. Personalized service conveys that you are a professional that genuinely cares about tailoring their care to their specific needs. Customized service is quality patient care, and the communication between the healthcare worker and the patient is improved.

The following **CARE** skills can help healthcare professionals improve professionalism and patient interactions. Caring for patients should be primary for all healthcare professionals and creating positive patient experiences can lead to patient satisfaction. Patient satisfaction measures the quality in health care. Patient satisfaction should be the focus on every person who works with or takes care of patients.

Ten Ways to Show Customers You Care

The CARE skills can improve a patient and health professional's relationship. The care skills can help healthcare practitioners demonstrate empathy and concern for patients. Healthcare workers provide high-quality service when they apply these skills.

Encourage customers to talk	Use empathy
Be attentive	Show appreciation
Convey respect	Show dignity
Ask for permission	Focus on the customer
Be polite	Use positive body language

Showing care and concern displays professionalism. It's important to speak to customers in a positive and accommodating manner. Showing customers courtesy is the first step in conveying care and concern.

Demonstrate your CARE concern

In a group role paly the care skills and discuss best practices in patient care.

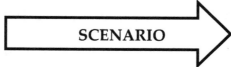

SCENARIO

Customer Service for Healthcare Professionals

What should happen to the employees in the scenario? How should Ms. Jackson be accommodated?

Ms. Jackson is a patient and comes to desk and signs in and claims to have an appointment, but it cannot be found in the electronic health record scheduling system. She states that a woman named Kristen scheduled her appointment. Kristen is a new employee and not too knowledgeable of the scheduling system and says that Kristen must have made a mistake. Ms. Jackson is angry because the waiting room is full of people and she has been waiting for 45 minutes while Chris a senior employee searches for her appointment. Ms. Jackson states that have taken off work today and needs to get to the dentist. Chris comes to you in a panic because he fears that he is on the verge of being fired and he does not want her to complain to the office manager.

1. Should you reschedule her appointment?
2. Should you fit in her the schedule?
3. Should Chris be fired?
4. Should Kristen be trained on the scheduling systems?
5. Should the office manager speak to Ms. Jackson?

Pair up and role-play a care quality.

Chapter 3

HIPAA – Protecting Health Information

HIPAA is the federal Health Insurance Portability and Accountability Act (HIPAA) of 1996. The primary goal of the law is to make it easier for people to protect the confidentiality and security of healthcare information. HIPAA is comprised of two overarching parts--the Privacy Rule and Security Rule.

The HIPAA Privacy Rule provides federal protections for personal health information and offers patients an array of rights concerning that information. At the same time, the Privacy Rule permits the disclosure of personal health information needed for patient care and other vital purposes. The Security Rule specifies a series of administrative, physical, and technical safeguards for covered entities to use to assure the confidentiality, integrity, and availability of electronic protected health information. (www.hhs.gov)

The following information regarding privacy and confidentiality can be located in a HIPAA training (www.hipaaclickandcomply.com)

What is Protected Health Information (PHI)?

PHI is information that is recorded in written records, and all communication and electronic media must be protected.

Customer Service for Healthcare Professionals

For example, if you are talking with the patient discussing health conditions on the phone, you must be careful that someone in your organization cannot get the information. Additionally, information that is on a computer or sent via fax must be protected. If you have a computer database of patient files, you must be sure that access to this information is limited. You must also be careful to protect data on your computer screen.

The organization maintains PHI's information that is either collected by your organization. For example, you may have a patient, previous medical record that you did not originate. You must protect these records. Information that is forwarded to someone else must also be protected. For example, if your office forward's the data to a billing agency to process your bills differently- this information must be protected. You also are required to ensure that the billing agency is keeping information secure as required by HIPAA.

PHI is information that identifies an individual or could identify an individual includes necessary information such as; the person's name, so security number, home address, phone number, and driver's license. However, it also includes less obvious information such as the place of employment, names of relatives, or physical descriptions (gender or hair color).

PHI is information that relates to the individual condition, treatment, or payment in the past, present, or future.

For example, a discussion of a patient's previous condition must also be protected. When you are discussing treatment with the patient, you must guarantee a secure setting which protects the patient's privacy.

How or when can PHI be used?

PHI can be used to disclose when patient consent authorization for treatment, payment, or health care operations.

Who is included as an employee, business association, or representative?

HIPAA requirements bind the following groups of persons; all employees who work with PHI in the course of meeting with their job description and medical professionals who provide direct healthcare or office support workforce members who record information. HIPAA law also requires business associate or representatives used by agencies in delivering services. One example, a doctor's office using a billing agency or laboratory for services would be included.

What does a patient need to know?

The patient needs to know who requested information, what they are seeking, why they are asking, and when they would like to receive it.

What is the penalty for HIPAA violations?

Protecting patient health information is very serious, and failure to comply HIPAA may result in penalties of $100 to $50,000 per violation, depending on the conduct at issue. If the violation results from "willful neglect" the party is subject to mandatory fines of $10,000 per violation with a maximum of $250, 000 for a repeat violation. The maximum is $50,000 per violation with an annual maximum of 1.5 million. According to Health and Human Services (HHS), a covered entity may avoid HIPAA penalties, if it does not act with "willful neglect" and corrects the violation within 30 days.

How to Avoid a HIPAA Violation

Policies and procedures that govern the use and disclosures of protected health information can minimize the risk of violations. In every instance of use or disclosure of protected health information employees must make judgments about the identity, role, authority, and need of each user/recipient based upon these judgments, we must then define the type and amount of public health information (PHI) the user/recipient will be able to have. In every instance, this means providing only the minimum PHA that is necessary for the user/recipient to perform their role with limited data; it must also be determined, if the patient's approval is required before the disclosure of protected health information, either within the organization or to outside individuals and other organizations.

For most companies the typical activities such as treatment, payment, and operations (TPO), judgments are made up front by establishing policies rather than on a case to case basis. These judgments will enable you to develop standards and practices and agreements that will allow a variety of activities in the workforce and among the workforce members to perform their duties without having to seek guidance in every instance.

For the use of disclosure circumstances that are not typical generally, not related to TPO, judgments must be made almost about almost every request. Therefore, the privacy officer at your organization should be involved in all atypical uses and disclosures.

Documentation must include all of the following in the body of a form before patient information is released.

1. The personal organization requesting the information

2. Purpose of the request for the PHI

3. Data requests

4. Description of the PHI disclosure

5. Date of the disclosure

Disclosing Information to Patients:

In most cases, patients have the right to see or obtain a copy of his or her information.

Disclosure of PHI to Other Providers:

If a request from another provider is a made or you have concerns about the legitimacy of the request, you should consult with your privacy officer, but always follow the established office procedures. However, make sure that the people requesting information are who they claim to be and have the authority to receive the PHI. Please review verification requirement procedures at your organization.

For Treatment:

If another provider is seeking PHI to treat a patient, you should not release any of the PHI without the patient's authorization. As a standard practice psychotherapy notes cannot be disclosed without a patient's consent.

Child Abuse:

Under HIPAA agencies can report suspicion of child abuse. Other laws may also require such disclosure; in this case, the privacy officer should preside over such disclosures. An agency may not be required to get an authorization agreement from the patient or, the represent when making such disclosures. In addition to necessary information about the PHI that is being disclosed a statement regarding patient notification of the PHI being at risks of being disclosed should be included. When the request is made, the recipient must indicate whether or, not the patient should receive the information about the disclosure. For example, if an investigation is being conducted, it may be appropriate for the disclosure of the PHI to be kept confidential from the patient.

Abuse, Neglect or Domestic Violence against an Adult:

As a standard practice you can disclose the minimum necessary PHI in adults or victims of abuse, neglect, or domestic violence to a social service authorized to receive such information under the following circumstances;

• Disclosures required by law.

• The disclosures allowed by statute or regulation and, in your professional judgment, you believe a disclosure necessary to prevent serious harm to the patient or other potential victims.

• The disclosures allowed by statute or regulation and, if the patient is unable to agree has been capacitive and capacitive, a public official (including law enforcement) agrees that PHI will not be used against the patient and also claims that waiting for patient consent would adversely affect related enforcement activities.

In regards to HIPAA (PHI) and The Affordable Care Act (ACA), employers should be sure the vendor is contractually bound to maintain and implement appropriate privacy and security practices. Employers must determine whether the information is subject to HIPAA. Employers need to consider whether this information collected for ACA group health plans and reporting requirements, is protected health information under HIPAA (PHI).

The employer needs to implement safeguards to ensure patient privacy and take appropriate steps under the HIPAA privacy and security rules. The HIPAA law requires that every doctor, hospital, or other health care providers provide the patient with a copy of the Notice of Privacy Practice. The Patient Rights under HIPAA protects the patient's healthcare information. Healthcare professionals can avoid

HIPAA violations, by complying with their healthcare organizations privacy practices.

Chapter 4

Building Customer Service Relationships

In healthcare greeting a patient by name is the best way to make them smile. Greeting customers are one of the most critical communication skills a healthcare professional can possess. A greeting is one of the primary functions that can cause positive conversations. We get to know people when we communicate with them. Greeting people helps us connect on a more personal level.

BEHAVIORAL INFLUENCE STAIRWAY

The Behavioral Change Stairway Model was developed by the FBI's hostage negotiation unit and shows the five steps to getting someone else to see your point of view and change what they're doing. The behavioral influence stairway can help you deal with hostile and angry patients. The five steps can help you work with difficult, angry, or furious patients and avoid misunderstandings. (www.fed.gov)

Active Listening: When you take time and listen to others you are showing concern.

Empathy: It is the ability to understand and share the feelings of others.

Rapport: Showing kindness and being friendly is essential in building rapport. Rapport building helps patients trust and open up to you.

Influence: Showing empathy and building a report can influence positive treatment outcomes.

Behavioral Change: How to act.

Every business has its share of upset and angry customers and, healthcare is no different. If you are providing a service or running a business, there are all types of customers. Illnesses affect patients physically, mentally and emotionally and they can get irate and become angry and frustrated. Communication and active listening are necessary skills to handle patient/customer concerns and complaints. For this reason, you need to document patient interactions and services provided. Problem-solving skills can help you minimize conflict, but they may not prevent a patient from filing a complaint. However, problem-solving skills can help create patient satisfaction. The overall goals in healthcare are to provide quality patient care and create positive, memorable experiences.

The five methods for building relationships can help you create positive patient experiences.

Five Methods to Building Customer

1. Smile with your greetings – Customers want to hear positive words and see a smile when greeted. We recommend that you say, "Hello, welcome to ____, how may I serve you? " Always say, good afternoon, good morning or good evening.

2. Introduce yourself- While you are smiling inform the customer of your name and position. For example, "Hello, my name is ____, I am a medical assistant, and how may I serve you? When greeting a customer use their name; for example, "Welcome, Mr. Miss, or Mrs. Brown how are you today?

3. Ask the question -You must ask the customer what they need and want. For example; if a patient is admitted to the hospital you may ask: Is there anything that I can do to make you comfortable? Is there anything that you feel you need? If you ask them, they will tell you.

4. Professional Dress - You will be the first person a patient will see, and first impressions are lasting. You want to have good hygiene. Comb your hair and brush your teeth daily. Dressing and acting professional is the perception that you set for your company. Women and men are encouraged to avoid strong cologne or

perfume. Healthcare professionals should cover all tattoos and body piercings. Most healthcare facilities require uniform conformity and should conform and wear uniforms and avoid provocative outfits.

5.   Know your customer needs, wants and expectations - To get to know your customer you must understand what your customer need, want and expect. It may apply to patients that have been admitted and treated at a hospital or a long-term care facility. Healthcare workers should confer with the physician, supervisor, or the director of nursing.

The following list of customer needs can help you efficiently and effectively serve patients.

Help

Someone to listen

Respect

A Smiling face

Quality service

Satisfaction

Honesty

A Knowledgeable Professional

Getting to know your patient/customer by name is essential in building a patient relations and long-lasting care healthcare relationship. Getting to know your customer can help promote quality care.

Ten Tips for Improving Customer Relationships

1. Greet patients with a smile

2. Get to know your patients

3. Know the company services

4. Determine the patients' needs

5. Meet the patients' needs

6. Know your company's policy on patient practices

7. Handle patient complaints professionally

8. Present solutions- Share what you can do

9. Send reminder notices or telephone calls

10. Follow- up with patients by phone or mail

Internal and External Relationships

Customer Service for Healthcare Professionals

External customers are a person who comes to the health care facility for help or provides a service for your company. External customer service is the way someone views your company and service. External customers could be the patient, relatives, companions, or representatives. Customer service is crucial to achieving any business success.

Internal customer service is an example of an employee and employer relationship. Recruiting, hiring and training the best employees can produce quality service. An internal customer would be a co-worker or a distributor who depends upon the company to provide products or services.

Everyone who works for the company or is a third party that provides products or services is a customer. All internal and external customers deserve the same level of customer service.

List 4 Ways to Improve Internal and External Customer Relations

Internal Customers Examples	External Customer Examples

Customer Follow-Up

As a standard practice, a post-healthcare follow-up should begin after each healthcare visit. Poor monitoring is one of patients/customer's biggest complaints. When a patient receives a call from their physician's office or medical facility, they feel cared for and valued. Healthcare professionals should follow- up and follow through on all commitments. A follow-up telephone call can be seen as good customer service and increase the organization's growth and profitability. A follow-up after a patient's release from the hospital is good customer service. However, if you contact the patient while they are in the hospital, this can be considered exceptional customer service.

Following- up with patients shows that you are serious and they are valued, and it can increase customer loyalty and retention. As a professional in healthcare, do not make promises that you cannot keep. Only promise what you know you can deliver. Following -up with patients is critical to compliance and outcomes, but can reduce healthcare risk and improve safety. Healthcare experts say that failing to follow-up with patients can lead to significant legal dangers for medical practices and healthcare organizations.

1. Give scenarios of best practices for ensuring effective follow-up

_____

_____

Chapter 5

The Patient Experience

Many healthcare professionals interact with patients before, after, and during office visits and hospital admissions. Several effective patient contact interactions will determine satisfaction; including the "hellos and goodbyes." One unfortunate customer service experience can turn a customer away. If a patient had a poor customer service experience on the telephone, that first impression could ruin the relationship. Each contact with a patient or the patient's representative is essential. The overall goals are to create positive, memorable experiences and make patients feel valued.

The following tips can improve a patient's customer experience.

1. Be helpful- usually, a disappointed patient tells 25 other people about the negative experience.

2. Be positive - For each patient who complains 20 other disappointed patients don't grumble. Research suggests that of those frustrated patients who don't complain, 10 percent will return while 90 percent won't.

3. Be authentic- show sincerity when greeting and helping customers.

The patient will have a positive customer service experience if shown concern and empathy. One of the essential customer service skills is communication. If you ask the right questions, you can find out how to meet patients' needs and provide quality care and exceptional customer service. Asking searching questions can help you to determine what the patient needs.

Four Step Process to Improve Patient Experience

1. Listen
2. Ask
3. Repeat
4. Present

Best Practices: Repeat what you heard to avoid any misunderstandings. For example, if a prescription was written and you cannot read it- clarify it with the medical provider to prevent a medical error.

Asking the following questions can help you determine and meet your patient/customer needs.

➢ How can I assist you today?
➢ What day and time would you like to schedule an appointment?

> ➢ How did you hear about us?
> ➢ What brought you here today?

Asking the list of questions can help you know if a patient/customer was satisfied or dissatisfied.

> ➢ How were you treated?
> ➢ Would you recommend our facility?
> ➢ What can we do to keep your business?
> ➢ What can we do better?
> ➢ Were you satisfied with your services?

The responses from these five questions can help you assess the changes that are needed. The importance of customer service surveys and follow-ups are essential to revenue and growth. Excellent customer service is linked to profitability just as comparable prices are too customer referrals. When customer /patient satisfaction and quality of care were provided, the healthcare workers meet the standard of excellent customer service.

Customer satisfaction surveys provide feedback and can help you poll customers and gather data. Customer service surveys help you evaluate how well you provided a service, how well the staff provided service, and how satisfied patients were with the service they received. Customer service comments and surveys can also be used to streamline how to improve efficiency and customer interaction.

Remember: Always to provide service with a smile

All customers want is to be heard and feel valued. Professionals who work in healthcare must learn to listen intently. Good listening is listening with the intent to understand and serve. Effective listening is an active process and necessary for understanding. Effective listeners maintain eye contact and understand that non-verbal communication is as important as verbal communication to avoid misunderstandings.

Are You a Good Listener?

Listening intently and clarifying the request or question can help you avoid any misunderstandings. Summarizing your customer's response and repeating patient request are useful methods to prevent any miscommunication. We always want to be professional and respectful when working with patients/customers.

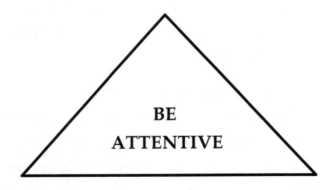

Customer Service for Healthcare Professionals

When you first meet a patient, you'll need to introduce yourself to make the patient feel at ease. Be attentive, considerate, and observant to understand and meet the patient's needs. Some patients are confused, nervous, and anxious when seeking medical attention. A friendly introduction to a patient /customer is essential in patient relations. For example: "Hello, Mr. Brown my name is Johnathan, I am your nurse and will be taking care of you today until 3 pm. If the patient is admitted into the hospital write your name on the whiteboard in their room. Inform that patient to press the call button, if they need your assistance.

Excellent customer service always wants to meet the needs of the customer. Once a patient gets to know you, and you address their needs and concerns they'll usually rate your service as outstanding.

The goal is to provide quality customer service that yields customer satisfaction.

The Five A's for the Customer's Checklist

- ❖ Acknowledge – the patient
- ❖ Affirm- the patient is in control of his or her healthcare
- ❖ Appreciate- something about working with the patient.
- ❖ Available –meet the patient needs

❖   Assure – the patient/customer is satisfied

Remember: If the patient is satisfied, everything else will follow.

You can provide effective customer service once you know what a patient needs. In healthcare, professionals are knowledgeable, and experts, and sometimes patients get angry when they don't know the answers. When you encounter a problem make sure that you know the person you can contact to answer patient questions and solve problems. We always want to resolve problems and patients complaints quickly and professionally.

The service goals are to provide high-quality patient care and create positive experiences to achieve patient satisfaction. Once a patient has received treatment or discharged, they usually receive a discharge survey or customer service survey via email. The customer feedback lets the organizations know what they are doing right and what changes need are needed. Always ask customers what they like about the medical facility or the healthcare provider.

Patient satisfaction surveys are utilized as indicators for measuring the quality in healthcare. Patient responses can help the administration make the necessary corrections and changes. Their feedback can improve service quality and patient relations.

There are words that every employee should use when working with customers. In healthcare, language is a caring skill that can change a patient's reaction, response and create positive experiences.

Customer Service for Healthcare Professionals

May I	I understand	May I help you?
I am delighted to	It is my pleasure	I am happy
Yes, we have this	Delighted	I apologize
I made a mistake	Happy	Which do you prefer?
Will you?	Yes	How can I help you?

Once, positive words are conveyed patients will usually respond appropriately. Healthcare professionals should use words that the patient can understand. Do not use medical jargon and medical terms that the patient cannot understand. Using caring language and kind words can build patient relations.

Pair up and use the five A's to create a patient and healthcare worker exchange using positive words and caring language.

1. _____
   _____
2. _____
   _____
3. _____
   _____
4. _____
   _____
5. _____

Chapter 6

Types of Customer Behaviors

Understanding customer behaviors will quickly tell you just how and what to say to each customer. Although every customer is different, they all have needs and concerns. Whether you're providing a service in a healthcare facility or running a business, you will come in contact with various types of personalities. The ten types of customer behaviors can help healthcare workers work with diverse people. When you learn to identify customer behaviors, you can exceed their expectations and provide exceptional customer service. Understanding and recognizing the customer behaviors can help healthcare professionals manage customer complaints and deliver excellent customer service.

Ten Types of Customer Behaviors

1. The Talkative Customer
2. The Dependent Customer
3. The Resistant Customer
4. The Complaining Customer
5. The Know It All Customer
6. The Satisfied Customer
7. The Angry Customer

8. The Inpatient Customer
9. The Rude Customer
10. The Hostile Customer

The ten types of customer behaviors can help healthcare professionals understand diverse types of customers. For example; if you have a talkative customer it's important to control the conversation. If you have an angry, impatient or rude or hostile customer- listen, be calm and be patient. Remember the customer may not be right, but the customer is a customer. Identifying the behavior and personality types of customers can help you emotionally self-regulate if a conflict arises. Healthcare professionals who understand the various types of customer behaviors can manage and handle customer complaints and solve problems more professionally.

Customer Service for Healthcare Professionals

Talkative	
Dependent	
Resistance	
Know It All	
Satisfied	
Angry	
Inpatient	
Rude	
Hostile	

Form a group and give an example of each type of customer behavior

Think like a Patient

There is an old saying, which I find to be true, *"treat others like you want to be treated."* Or better than that, **"treat them like family."**

Use positive words in a sentence to describe how you would like to treated as a patient.

You can create a positive patient experience if you treat patients like you want to be treated. The key phrase: **"What can you do to create a positive patient experience?"**

What Can You Do?

List 3 ways you can create positive patient experiences and provide superior customer service. Taking care of patients is what healthcare is all about.

The list of ten things that customers need can help you provide superior customer service. It is essential to practice these in your interactions with customers routinely. Practice will make them a part of your attitude and behavior.

Ten things can improve patient outcomes.

1. Empathy- Listen to their needs

2. Help- Offer assistance

3. Kindness-A friendly attitude

4. A smiling face- Is a friendly face

5. Patience - Compassion

6. Understanding- Reasonable

7. A quality product-

8. Support – Feeling of acceptance

9. Appreciation- Always says "thank you."

10. Respect- You care

Empathy is a critical skill in healthcare and sharing empathy is an essential component for human contact. Sharing compassion is one way of providing support. It is never wrong to let a patient know that you're trying to understand them from their frame of reference.

Share the difference between empathy and sympathy and answer question. Should you ever tell a patient, "I know how you feel?" If not why!

Empathy	Sympathy
Feeling the same emotions as the other person	Feeling sorrow or concern for the other person

Customer Service for Healthcare Professionals

Pair up and create a patient exchange and use the skill empathy. Share the difference between empathy and sympathy.

Should you ever tell a patient, "I know how you feel?" If not why!

_____

_____

Empathy	Sympathy

Chapter 7

Communication Skills in Healthcare

A customer's choice of words, the tone of voice and rate of speed may tell you something about his or her needs and expectations. The term communication is "the exchange of information (a message) between two or more people." Communication skills are verbal and non-verbal words, phrases, voice tones, facial expressions, gestures, and body language is used in the interaction between you and another person. According to the Webster dictionary verbal communication "is the behavior and elements of speech aside from the words themselves that transmit meaning."

Non-verbal communication includes "pitch, speed, tone, and volume of voice, gestures and facial expressions, body posture, stance, and proximity to the listener, eye movements and contact, and dress and appearance." (www.businessdictionary).

Written communication should be clear and legible.

Oral communication is the ability to exhibit essential listening and non-verbal communication skills. Accurate communication can improve patient/customer exchanges and prevent medical errors.

Communication Skills

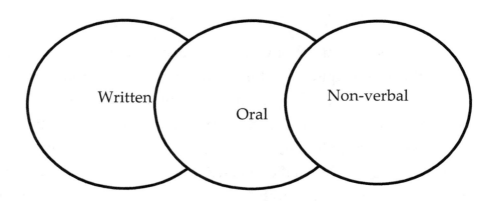

Oral Communication: Presentation, Body Language, Effective Listening

Written: Presentation, Reading and Documentation

Non-Verbal Communication: Body language, Presentation

Effective communication is a part of building and maintaining good physician-patient and nurse-patient relationships. These skills help professional healthcare workers provide exceptional customer service. Excellent communication skills are critical in healthcare, whether it is face-to-face, over the phone, via email or through online channels. Clear communication can build internal and external relationships and can help to avoid any misunderstandings.

Customer Service for Healthcare Professionals

Healthcare professional should communicate the medical instructions to patients clearly, and encouraged them to follow their doctor's instructions. Persuasive communication can help healthcare professional's influence patients to take better care of their health. Healthcare professionals can use patient education programs to help patients improve wellness. Good communication is vital in working with patients/customers in healthcare.

Communication skills are essential and helpful in developing a good relationship with other people. Quality care and excellent interpersonal skills are critical in retaining loyal patients/customers. If you apply the techniques and strategies in this book, you can improve your communication and active listening skills. Customer satisfaction can lead to patient referrals, patient retention, and positive patient/customer experiences.

Good communication demonstrates that you are professional and poor communication indicates that you are unprofessional. In healthcare, a connection is a key to providing quality patient care. Being proficient in contact helps you connect with patients, co-workers, superiors, and internal and external customers. Clear communication and active listening has a place in all human interactions. In healthcare, good communication can prevent medical errors. An effective communicator focuses entirely on the patient, their body language, and other nonverbal cues. Patients want to have quality interactions with healthcare professionals, and therefore, when they are talking, we need to show empathy and have patience.

Customer Service for Healthcare Professionals

Once you have developed proficient communication skills, it should become a part of your everyday communication style. Active listening to patients is crucial in showing them that you care. A healthcare worker on the road to proficiency should practice on improving his or her listening and communicating skills. As noted, communication is a direct reflection of the patient's perception of you as a professional. An excellent communicator connects with the patient/customer on an emotional level. For example, if a customer is angry or frustrated, you could say, "I hear that you are angry and you feel frustrated. I will work to solve your concern." Acknowledging a customer's feeling and demonstrates empathy, and is a mild form of social influence. A simple, cordial response to a customer's concern or complaint can shift emotions from angry to happy.

Both verbal and nonverbal are forms of communication. In healthcare, we encounter people of different ethnicities and cultures. Amazingly, people across all cultures understand the value of a smile which is non-verbal communication. Once you have developed proficient communication skills, it should become a part, of your everyday communication style. Good communication helps to decrease misunderstandings and build good relationships. A healthcare professional on the road to proficiency should practice, on improving his/ her listening and communication skills. Good communication is the key to solving- problems, decreasing conflicts, and maintaining relationships.

Customer Service for Healthcare Professionals

A smile shows that you are approachable and friendly. Friendliness is a basic expectation of employees who that in healthcare. Smiling, appearing approachable, and saying, "thank you" are exceptional customer service skills. Healthcare professionals should be patient and courteous to customers who are seeking medical attention. Healthcare professionals that "go the extra mile" can be seen as providing exceptional customer service. Positive customer service feedback can lead to a promotion, pay increase or a service award. Customer feedback allows healthcare facilities to measure how satisfied customers are with their service. The overall goals of an organization are to provide quality healthcare and customer satisfaction. Customer feedback allows your company to make the proper adjustments to improve service and quality of care. The overall goals of the healthcare industry are to provide quality services and products. The central goals in customer service are to build relationships, ensure quality care, and satisfy customers.

Satisfied customers tell other people about their customer experience. Exceptional customer service can improve customer satisfaction and have a positive impact on a business. Any businesses, churches, or political organizations can benefit from excellent customer service. If customers know that you care they will tell others about their experience. Customer satisfaction surveys provide feedback and help you poll customers and gather data. Good communication is vital in retaining patients/customers, avoiding medical errors, and gaining new ones. Someone once said, "Customer satisfaction is one of the best advertisements, and it cost nothing."

Customer Service Telephone Etiquette

In telephone customer service connecting with and understanding is one of the most important, and often most challenging stage in serving customers, because it requires you to concentrate entirely on what the patient is saying. A healthcare worker who focuses on the customer at the initial stage concentrates on everything the patient/customer is saying. Not only the words themselves, but the tone and how they speak to a patient shows appreciation of, and concern for, the customer's feelings and needs.

In some situations, you may find yourself holding only a brief conversation with the patient/customer. Whatever position you may find yourself in, you must concentrate on the patient/customer as an individual. Healthcare is patient-centered and professionals respectfully respond to, individual's preferences and needs.

The skills you need to understand the patient/customer;

- ❖ active listening for feelings and facts
- ❖ asking questions to clarify
- ❖ restating feelings and facts
- ❖ observe patients
- ❖ review medications
- ❖ write legible
- ❖ do not use white

- ❖ double check procedure
- ❖ follow procedures

Effective Listening

Form a group and provide examples of what you can do to avoid medical errors on the telephone or in person.

Listening to the feelings and facts as stated by patients, is critical to maintaining a positive interaction, building trust and confidence. Trust, effective communication, active listening, and consistency can create patient/customer satisfaction. Developing effective communication and listening skills are crucial in managing and solving customer concerns and problems. Listening requires a significant amount of concentration especially in situations in which the customer is difficult or upset. Active listening helps to avoid or lessen misunderstandings. Listening requires that you are open-minded and maintain direct eye contact at the speaker. (Unless direct eye contact is culturally disrespectful)

Smiling and maintaining eye contact are both critical in active listening. A smile shows customers that you are friendly and approachable. Communication is the most crucial skill in the healthcare industry. The lists of telephone dos and don'ts can help healthcare professionals interact more professionally with patients/customers.

Pair up and create and solve a patient's problems, i.e. appointment or medication

TELEPHONE SKILLS; Do's and Don'ts

Do	Don't
Take the caller's name early	Forget who you are talking to
Use their name often	Become distracted by people or things
Smile while you dial	
Stay in control by asking questions	Sound depressed
	Let the customer take control of call
Take notes while on the telephone	Talk for 15 seconds without asking a question
Pay attention and show that you are listening	Talk more than the customer-talk to fast
Be sincere	Slouch in your seat
Be enthusiastic	Be rude or sarcastic
Be friendly	Put people on hold without asking
Adjust your voice so you are not talking to loud	their permission
Answer within 3 to 5 rings	Put people on hold for longer than
Know how to use your phone hold and transfer	30 seconds, without going back to the
Always say " please" and " thank you	Cover the mouthpiece to talk to someone else. Use a whole button
Give information clearly	assume anything – check for
Summarize what has been agreed upon	understanding
	Put the telephone down before the customer does

Chapter 8

Handling Customer Complaints

Solving customer complaints are an opportunity to turn dissatisfied customers into satisfied customers. The following methods and techniques are designed to help healthcare professionals solve problems and handle irate customers. First, every employee should develop skills to address customer complaints effectively and appropriately. Resolving customer complaints should be resolved quickly. Second, employees should develop skills to self-regulate their emotions to handle and manage customer complaints professionally. Lastly, developing active listening skills and verbal, written, and oral communication skills can minimize conflict and avoid misunderstandings.

The 16 positive words are used in healthcare to maximize customer satisfaction.

- Clarity
- Honesty
- Kindness
- Efficiency
- Knowledgeable
- Understanding
- Gentleness
- Respectful
- Thoughtfulness
- Quality

Customer Service for Healthcare Professionals

- Prudence
- Soft-spoken
- Blessed
- Considerate
- Empathy
- Thank You
- Adequate

The acronym for **R.E.S. P.E.C.T** describes the behavior a healthcare professional should possess to improve patient satisfaction.

Respond: Be attentive and actively listen.

Engage: Handle and resolve problems promptly.

Support: Be courteous, kind and smile.

Professional: Be respectful and helpful.

Empathy: Show concern.

Communicate: Listen carefully and repeat what you heard in the conversation.

Communications: Communication is a key part of building a healthy patient and practitioner relationship. Respectful discussion is considered professional. If you tell a patient that you are going to schedule an appointment or send a referral, keep your word.

Problem Solving: The following is the systemic approach to problem-solving.

> 1. Define the problems
>
> 2. Gather Data
>
> 3. Review solutions
>
> 4. Select solutions
>
> 5. Monitor results

The problem-solving strategy **RESOLVE** reinforces the systemic approaches to resolving issues-

R. E. S. O. L.V.E

Repeat: To gain a better understanding of what you heard a person say, you should repeat the information to clear up any misunderstanding.   Rephrasing can clarify what was said.

Examine: Body language and voice tones are an integral part of problem-solving. Use non-threatening body language and calm voice tones to de-escalate conflicts and prevent workplace violence incidents.

Simplify: State and identify the current problem. Stay focused on the issue, and behavior. If performance problems exist follow personnel policies. Report and document all incidents.

Customer Service for Healthcare Professionals

Openly: Communicate openly and respectfully. Be a good listener and allow the employee or patient to share their thoughts on assigned task or ideas.

List: Write your goals and review weekly and monthly performance goals.

Validate: Be open to feedback without judging it as good or bad. Validate and acknowledge the patient, person, manager of co-worker opinion or observation.

Evaluate: Body language, voice tones, and behaviors are forms of communication. New responses can help a healthcare professional or leader find new ways to problem-solve. Be open-minded, flexible, and open to change.

Communication techniques and problem-solving strategies can improve human relations and de-escalate a hostile, angry customer/patient. Developing problem-solving skills can be personally and professionally beneficial.

Form a group and create a problem and find a solution to improve customer satisfaction.

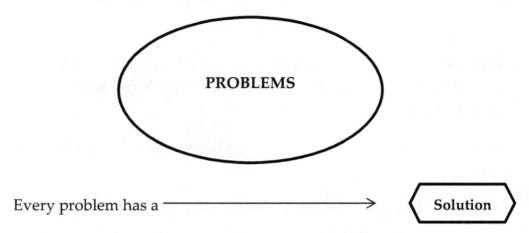

Every problem has a ⟶ ⟨ Solution ⟩

Form a group and create a problem and find solutions.

Problem	Solution

What could you or should you have done differently?

Form a group and create a problem and a solution.

Chapter 9

Professional Workplace Behaviors

Poor workplace performance can cause a business to lose customers and employees to lose jobs. The customer is the lifeblood of any business and professionalism now plays a much more critical role in the healthcare industry. Professionalism is a mindset, and those who possess it are much more likely to reap the rewards of success. If you are a new employee to a healthcare facility, you will receive an orientation package an employee and book. The information informs you about your position and includes, a mission statement, professional code of conduct, ethical codes, policies, and procedures and professional workplace behaviors such as; appearance, communication, body language, and attitude. Selling, soliciting, imposing religious and political beliefs on company time is unprofessional and could be against company policy.

A healthcare worker that is competent will adhere to policies and procedures in professional workplace behaviors. Research suggests uniformity in healthcare influences self-image and professional identity. In the ultra-competitive twenty-first century, you need more than medical credentials to advance in the healthcare industry. Companies are now putting a much greater emphasis on other employee attributes such as; professionalism, people skills, customer service skills, leadership capabilities, and team building abilities.

Professionalism is the culmination of competence, attitude, knowledge, interpersonal skills and how you work with others. Professionalism in the workplace can benefit your career and improve your working environment. Understanding how to develop your effective work habits can improve professionalism. Working on your attitude and workplace behaviors can improve professionalism.

What is professionalism?

1. A specific behavior in the healthcare

2. Standards and professional roles

3. Demonstrated in our behavior

Healthcare professionals display the competency skills and professional workplace behaviors.

> Professionalism is a mindset, and specific behaviors should be evidence.
> Professionalism is evidence of our behavior in the workplace.
> Professionalism is providing high quality in healthcare.

Customer Service for Healthcare Professionals

What does the word "professionalism" mean to you? Take a moment to write down your definition.

_____

_____

_____

_____

_____

Identify three professional workplace behaviors

_____

_____

_____

Form a group and discuss positive workplace behaviors. Write down your responses. (Role-play the behaviors).

1._____

2._____

3._____

Customer Service for Healthcare Professionals

Professionalism has a lot to do with your values, how you act and communicate with others. Professionalism is displayed in the way healthcare professionals conduct themselves in professional situations. As a professional you have a demeanor that is courteous and polite when dealing with internal and external customers.

Internal Customers is an employee and employer relationship. Internal customers would be co-workers, peers, and superiors who work in the same company.

How can you improve internal customer satisfaction?

_____

External customers are insurance companies, healthcare providers, and customers from outside the company, or they receive products or services from the company. External customers pay for the service that the company provides.

How can you improve external customer satisfaction?

_____

Understanding the different kinds of people and personality types can help you successfully work with internal and external customers. There are several kinds of people in the world in which we live, the Striver, the Maintainer, the Struggler, and the Succeeder.

For the Striver:
- Provide specific direction.
- Give detailed instructions.

- Provide specific goals and objectives.
- Check frequently on their progress.
- Demonstrate steps to accomplishing a job.
- Enforce policies and conformity to methodologies.
- Channel the person's energy and motivation by providing structure and necessary training.

Use the description and provide an example of the behavior and action of a Striver.

For the Struggler:

- Convince the individual of her/his own ability to learn the job.
- Take time to listen and understand his/her situation, difficulties, and desires.
- Provide specific direction.
- Give detailed instructions.
- Provide particular goals and objectives.
- Demonstrate steps to accomplishing a job.
- Enforce policies and conformity to methodologies.

Use the description and provide an example of the behavior and action of a Struggler.

For the Maintainer

- Involve the individual in decisions that affect her/his work.
- Take time to listen and understand his/her situation, difficulties and desires, without criticizing or judging.
- Focus on obtaining the individual's support for projects and tasks.
- Solicit his/her input into work planning and task assignments.

Use the description and provide an example of the behavior and action of a Maintainer.

_____

For the Succeeder:

- Delegate broader responsibilities and let her/him handle the details.
- Encourage risk-taking and innovation, and provide feedback on results.
- Expect the individual to correct his or her errors.

Use the description and provide an example of the behavior and action of a Succeeder.

_____

Understanding and identifying the kinds of people, not only helps you work well with others, but improves your professional performance.

From the 4 kinds of people who are you?

What kind of person would you like to be?

What do you need to change to be the person you want to be?

Professionalism communicates to your internal and external customers that you have the knowledge, expertise, or background to deliver them quality service.

What can you improve professionally?

What can you do to stop letting your personal issues impact your professional life?

Professional development goals can help you expand your skills. Cross-departmental training can improve your career opportunities. Goal setting helps you obtain what they want in life.

The following steps are the processes to help you advance professionally and create career opportunities.

1. **Develop goals**
2. **Act on your ideas**
3. **Rely on your intuition**

4. Enjoy what you do

We are all unique people, and the acronym care can help you develop and fulfill your short and long-term career goals. Goals setting can help you accomplish your goals and advance professionally.

Six Month- Four Year Goals (short)	Five -Ten Year Goals (long)

Personal and Professional Goals

Customer Service for Healthcare Professionals

A personal self-improvement plan can improve your personal and professional life. What do you need to change to be an exceptional person?

Long and short-range goals setting can guide your life.

List three short range goals. (6 months - 1 year) (1-4 years)

1. _____

_____

2. _____

_____

3. _____

_____

Three long range goals (5-10 years)

1. _____

_____

2. _____

_____

3._____

The method of SMART goals is the acronym for the five steps to goal setting.

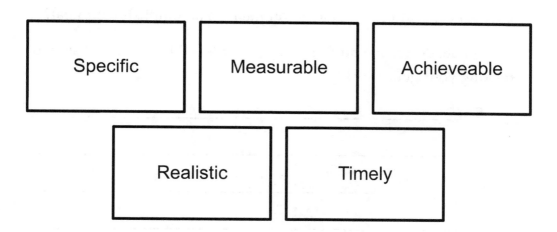

A goal helps you achieve what you want. A goal helps you achieve what you want. Every person should also set professional and personal goals to guide their life. The process of goal setting begins with first setting long-term professional goals. Next, start taking action. Last, monitor progress at each set benchmark or milestone.

Take a moment to write out one professional goal. Use the **SMART** acronym to work on developing a goal.

Are you moving forward towards a goal or stuck in procrastination? Most successful people who accomplish their goals are disciplined, motivated, and optimistic.

When you begin to set a goal to ask yourself what you want to accomplish. Next, what will you do differently to achieve your goal? Lastly, how will you be held accountable to accomplish your goal?

Write down one professional goal: **SMART** - is the first step to making your goal a reality.

S _____

M _____

A _____

R _____

T_____

Identify barriers that hinder you from reaching your goals.

Goals	Barriers

Customer Service for Healthcare Professionals

Methods to overcome barriers

_____

_____

_____

_____

Identify time frames to accomplish goals

_____

_____

_____

Identify barriers to excellent customer service.

Working with challenging and irate patients/customers is the leading cause of stress in the workforce. Often, the adverse effects of stress include illness, absenteeism, and alcohol abuse. Most employers have an employee assistance program (EAP) or, a wellness program to improve wellness. The following stress management strategies can help you bring your life into balance. It can be frustrating and challenging to balance work, family, and school. Time management and discipline can help you meet life's demands and obligations

Reminder: Goal setting is designed to motivate and guide you to achieve what you want. Time management, discipline, and organization skills help you reach your goals.

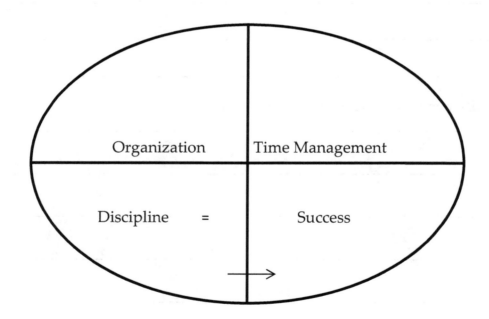

The following stress management techniques can provide you with a positive mental attitude and a feeling of well-being.

> ➢ Exercise
> ➢ Journaling (write down thoughts and feelings)
> ➢ Meditating
> ➢ Deep breaths
> ➢ Listening to music
> ➢ Laughing
> ➢ Drinking tea

With a busy life, time management and discipline can help you meet life's demands and obligations. The stress management techniques can help you be a happy, healthy, active, and productive employee.

Building Professional Relationships

With Co-Workers

- Be a team player
- Be flexible
- Greet coworkers and supervisors and customers
- Help others complete their task
- Do whatever it takes to get the job done

With Supervisor

- Don't miss deadlines
- Be timely
- Work hard
- Volunteer for assignments
- Be willing to take on new assignments
- Be honest and show respect
- Show a positive attitude

With a Healthcare Team

Within healthcare, each level of competency is identified to enhance effective teamwork. Teams in health care take many forms. For example, there are hospital teams, disaster response teams, physician group teams, and office-based care teams and teams that perform operations in hospitals.

The team building approach **STAR.** The acronym stands for S-Strategic Planning T- Team Approach A – Accountability/Access R-Relationships.

The **STAR** components are essential in building effective teams and goals and objections to team building projects.

S- Strategic Planning

1. Allowed members to develop teams and goals.
2. Identify components to produce a quality program project.
3. Establish action plans to meet goals.

Customer Service for Healthcare Professionals

T- Team Approach

1. Identify what processes are and are not effective and addresses areas that need   improvement.
2. Identify problems in their workplace poor performance and conflicts in groups.
3.   Identify areas that need improvement.

A - Accountability/Access

1. Identify team leaders, timelines, milestones, and benchmarks.
2. Take responsibility for your actions and results.
3. Identify staff skills and abilities to improve the quality and effectiveness.
4. Identify the people in the chain of command and organization structure.
5. Increase communication portals, i.e. access, e-mails, webinars,
6. Identify cross-training and cross-functional needs to increase productivity.

R- Relationships (Internal and External)

Internal relationships

1. Identify meeting dates and times; follow up with e-mails.
2. Identify team member's goals and relationship correlations.
3. Identify the working knowledge of the organization.
4. Developed cost matrix and departmental budgets to monitor revenue.

External relationships

1. Network to improve partnerships by gathering data to meet identified needs.
2. Advertise to improve visibility, grow revenue, and get new customers.

An effective healthcare team requires committed team members to fulfill the goals and objectives. The acronym **STAR** provides principles can help team members become unified so they can and complete projects. Team performance can lead to salary increases, bonuses, and termination.

Healthcare Professional Workplace Best Practices

Time Management

Time management is crucial in accomplishing specific tasks, projects, and goals. A person that is organized and manages their time wisely can achieve goals and exceed expectations. Time management, organizational skills, and a team player attitude can help you develop a strong professional image.

Time Management

- Develop weekly plans of what you need to accomplish.

- Prioritize the tasks according to the level of importance.
- Arrive at your work early and to meditate and get some quite
- Buy and use a day-planning calendar or system.
- Go through our inbox at least once a day and prioritize the contents.

Organizational Skills

- Keep your desk organized and clutter free
- Use your calendar to plan and manage appointments and meetings
- Develop an effective filing system
- Know how to use a computer

Voicemail Best Practices

- Let the caller know your name and that you will return the telephone call within 24 hours.
- Let the caller know the date, how and when they can reach you
- Informed the caller, if in the event you do not return their call within 24 hours that she should contact another person. So you should provide the name and telephone number of that person.

Email Best Practices

- Use the Subject line to capture attention with 50 words or less. Keep your message brief. Try to keep your line length at 50 characters or less. If your message is likely to be forwarded, keep it to 30 or less.

- Use the Standard English language (no- slang or text. Jargon) . Proofread every Email before hitting the send button.
- Avoid discussing private concerns and issues.
- Do not wait until the end of the day to introduce a problem or concern
- Be professional and respectful

Established limits that allow for safe connection between employees, patients, suppliers, and customers are professional. Creating healthy boundaries is an excellent way to keep your relationships professional.

Relationships: Good working relationships with others in a professional circle include patients/customers, suppliers, coworkers, peers, supervisors, and key stakeholders. It is essential to build and maintain good relations with these people.

The employee handbook presents the policies, procedures, and professional conducts. Employees are encouraged to reread the company's policies and procedures periodically. The lack of policy and procedure knowledge can lead to poor performance evaluation and employment termination.

The following list can lead to a negative employee performance evaluation or employment termination.

1. A violation of company policy

2. A repetitive pattern of absenteeism or tardiness

3. A person who is behaving unprofessionally

4. A person not responding well to feedback

5. A person who is not improving after a performance evaluation

Most organizations tie raises, bonuses, and compensation on employee performance reviews. If an employee receives an unsatisfactory performance, he or she may be required to correct behavior and work with a team. Sometimes, supervisors may need employees to be a part of a cross-functional team, and or be cross-trained. Cross-functional teams are useful when people from different departments and with diverse expertise come together to solve problems, and create innovative ideas and develop new approaches to improve quality. Cross-functional training and customer service training can help employees' function effectively and efficiently.

Healthcare professionals should be aware of their professional image in the workplace. Appearance, communication and body language, can create a more polish self-image. Honesty, integrity, and ethics are characteristics that professionals demonstrate in their personal life and workplace. Personal growth and development, high self-esteem, motivation, and respect are the benefits of professionalism. Common courtesy, customer focus, and respect represent the highest standards of healthcare professionals.

Chapter 10

Customer Service Activities

In healthcare, patient satisfaction is linked to outstanding customer service. Professionalism in customer service is the highest standard of quality. Quality customer service matters! Researchers report when customers are asked what makes a great customer experience they usually mention, something about genuineness, uniqueness, and a human touch. The customer service activities and assessments prepare healthcare professionals to handle just about any situation. The customer service activities, assessments, and group activities offer a hand on approach to teaching and learning for allied health students and those who work in the healthcare industry.

Defining Excellent Customer Service
Definition:
Neutral customers are those that had a nice, but not a memorable experience.

Satisfied customers are those who have a memorable experience and share those experiences with others.

Dissatisfied customers are those whose experience is less than their expectations. They will use negative words to describe their experience and share their experience with others.

Customer Service for Healthcare Professionals

Task

Work in a group and identify some actions and strategies that relate to each of the three experiences, using real-life examples if possible or, develop a patient experience.

Satisfaction	Dissatisfaction	Neutral

CUSTOMER SERVICE; True or False

Direction: Consider each of the following statements carefully and mark each with an X is either true or false

Statement	True	False
Follow up on customer experiences can increase loyalty		
The customer is always right		
In most organizations, good customer service training saves money		
The best way to measure of customer satisfaction is by customer complaints		
A customer that experiences dis-atisfaction is likely to tell others		
The customer that expense satisfaction will tell everyone		
Customer service training improves performance.		
Customers complain because they want good service		
It is difficult to tell if a customer satisfied		
A satisfied customer will become a loyal customer		

TELEPHONE SKILLS: True or False

Check true or false

Statement	True	False
It is best to answer the telephone on the 5th ring		
People like to be placed on hold		
It is best to speak fast so can answer another call quickly		
It is best never to keep the customer on hold for more than 4 minutes		
You should always address the customer by Mr. or Mrs.		
It is best to answer the telephone quickly		
You should answer you should address the customer by his or her first name because it makes you appear more friendly		

Happy Customers are Loyal Customers

HAPPY CUSTOMER

Directions: Describe as many words as you can from the following happy customers or write words that describe a happy customer.

KEY TELEPHONE SKILLS: Do's and Don'ts

Directions: Using the following the two columns below complete your own list of do's and don'ts.

Do's	Don'ts

COMMUNICATION SELF- ASSESSMENT

Directions: Complete the following questionnaire honestly. Rate your responses to each of the following

1= Never   2 = Sometimes   3 = Usually   4 =   Seldom   5 = Always

I communicate well with coworkers, patients, and supervisors.	1-2-3-4-5
I am considered a communication expert	1-2-3-4-5
I do not blame others for my mistakes	1-2-3-4-5
I use words negative words when speaking patients	1-2-3-4-5
In communication, I focus on hearing the patients problem	1-2-3-4-5
I use written and verbal communication well	1-2-3-4-5
I often explain something several times when I'm speaking to people	1-2-3-4-5
I get frustrated when I repeat myself	1-2-3-4-5
When upset I talk about others	1-2-3-4-5
I observe people's body language when communicating	1-2-3-4-5
I don't make other people feel stupid when giving feedback	1-2-3-4-5

ATTITUDE SELF -ASSESSMENT

1= Never   2 = Sometimes 3 = Usually   4 =   Seldom   5 = Always

Directions: Complete the following questionnaire. Rate your responses to each of the following.

I look so I look forward to learning something new every day	1-2-3-4-5
I am positive and optimistic about life	1-2-3-4-5
I compliment others whenever it is possible and I avoid criticism and gossip	1-2-3-4-5
I envy others co-workers and friends	1-2-3-4-5
The first thing I do is greet others in the workplace	1-2-3-4-5
I try to be well-dressed and groom to make me feel better	1-2-3-4-5
I do not get enough rest	1-2-3-4-5
I make a list of all the positive things I have done and how I did them	1-2-3-4-5
I believe when I make happens for other life makes happened for me	1-2-3-4-5
I believe that all hard work brings increase and benefits	1-2-3-4-5
I believe I am overweight	1-2-3-4-5
I strive to see the good in others	1-2-3-4-5
I know that most joy comes from enjoying the work and not reaching the stars	1-2-3-4-5

PROFESSIONAL ASSESSMENT

Take this assessment to evaluate your current level of professionalism.

I avoid criticizing a fellow co-worker. Yes   Sometimes   No
When meeting someone for the first time, I extend a firm handshake. Yes   Sometimes   No
I am considered a leader and role model for others Yes   Sometimes No
I warmly greet all of my co-workers each day.   Yes   Sometimes   No
I avoid discussing politics or religion at work Yes   Sometimes   No
I avoid discussing the performance of one employee with another employee.   Yes   Sometimes   No
I avoid criticizing a fellow co-worker in front of other co-workers. Yes   Sometimes   No
I am often late for work. Yes   Sometimes   No
I read the employee handbook often. Yes   Sometimes   No
I dress appropriately at work. Yes   Sometimes   No
I present a positive attitude at work at all times   Yes   Sometimes   No
I gossip about patients and coworkers Yes   Sometimes   No

PROFESSIONAL ASSESSMENT

Take this assessment to evaluate your current level of professionalism

I display a professional image at work.   Yes   Sometimes   No
I communicate clearly   Yes   Sometimes   No
I avoid contributing to company gossip.   Yes   Sometimes   No
I speak negatively about my employer and company   Yes   Sometimes   No
I always use correct grammar when speaking to others   Yes   Sometimes   No
I avoid using slang or sloppy language.   Yes   Sometimes   No
I always pay attention to the customer's facial expression and body language Yes   Sometimes   No
I avoid using slang language at work Yes   Sometimes   No
I am always positive and optimistic   Yes   Sometimes   No
I smile frequently when I am speaking with people.   Yes   Sometimes   No
I maintain appropriate eye contact with people when I speak to people Yes   Sometimes   No
I get along with people at work, if I don't like them Yes   Sometimes   No
I am very good at making small talk with almost anyone.   Yes   Sometimes   No

ATTITUDE

When you communicate your attitude shows. Building a rapport and relationship with customers begins with a positive attitude. Maintaining a positive attitude when dealing with difficult customers can be challenging, but it is essential in the hospitality industry.

A positive attitude can make an enormous impact on your customer relationship. Remaining positive when things are good is easy, but staying positive during difficult times is the challenge. If you can keep a positive attitude in all situations your life will become happier and successful.

When someone is displaying a negative attitude, what do you think about that individual?

_____

_____

_____

What can you do to have a more positive attitude during difficult times?

_____

_____

_____

Customer Service for Healthcare Professionals

Conclusion

Customer Service Training for Healthcare Instructor Manual provides methods and techniques to improve customer service practices and professional workplace behaviors for healthcare workers. The communication techniques and conflict resolution skills help students and employees resolve complaints appropriately and improve patient-centered care.

The program based learning provides independent learning, encourages brainstorming and team building approaches. The learning approach is based on adults and is student-centered that is interactive, relevant, and practical in the healthcare industry. Healthcare workers develop critical skills to provide excellent customer service that affects patient satisfaction.

The group activities, ongoing self-assessment, and customer service questionnaires reinforce the customer service principles and techniques. The healthcare techniques and strategies help healthcare professionals create positive patient experiences and customer satisfaction. Healthcare professionals learn to effectively communicate, greet patients, schedule appointments, and work in healthcare teams. Customer Service Training for Healthcare Professionals is written in English and Spanish to help students better communicate with their patients. Customer service training helps you learn specific knowledge and skills to improve patient care and patient/customer satisfaction.

Customer Service for Healthcare Professionals

Remember the Golden Rule

Treat Others Like You Want To Be Treated

Customer Service for Healthcare Professionals

About the Author

Reba Haley began her career at Allied Health by attending a medical assistant program and became a certified medical assistant. She worked as a medical assistant and office manager for years. She worked in hospitals, long-term care centers, and clinics as a nursing assistant, coordinator of the health unit and phlebotomist. Reba continued her education and attended a licensed practical nursing program. She graduated from the University of North Carolina with a degree in Psychology, obtained a Master of Science in Addiction Counseling, has extensive academic studies in Family and Marriage Therapy, and has a Doctorate in Counseling. She is a Registered Marriage and Family Therapist, Substance Abuse Professional and Certified Addiction Professional.

Professional, and performs drug and alcohol evaluations, and follow-up evaluations for employees who violate the Department of Transportation's drug and alcohol policy. Dr. Haley has years of experience working as an Instructor, Clinical Supervisor and Allied Health Officer in public schools and postsecondary schools. She is the President of Insight Consulting International Group, a business consulting firm that specializes in the development of customized training for corporations. Reba spent her entire professional career in business development, training, and advising. She is a life coach and conducts seminars, training, and workshops on customer service, leadership development, diversity, problem- solving, and relationship building techniques. She is the author of several training and self-improvement books travels conducting conferences within the United States and on board.

She is the founder and CEO of the New Beginnings Addiction and Wellness Center, a non-profit, tax-exempt organization in Florida, established to provide treatment for youth, adults, pregnant mothers, and youth that need treatment for opioids and other drugs. The agency offers a variety of human services and uses holistic and traditional treatment approaches to treat the disease of addiction. Her clinical history focused on the treatment of families, pregnant women, adolescents, and adults with concurrent disorders (addiction and mental illness). She is a specialist in addictions in the treatment of addiction and works with Steve Arkin, M.D. OB / GYN, and addiction consultant.

References

Office of Labor Statistics
https://www.bls.gov/ooh/healthcare/home.htm

Merriam and Webster Dictionary https://www.merriamwebster.com/

The Joint Commission https://www.jointcommission.org

The National Center for Health Statistics
https://www.cdc.gov/nchs/index.htm

The National Coordinator of Health Information Technology
https://www.healthit.gov/topic/health-it-basics/benefits-ehrs

CPSIA information can be obtained
at www.ICGtesting.com
Printed in the USA
LVHW022240151220
674262LV00006B/339